Crisis and Growth: Helping Your Troubled Child

CHARLOTTE H. and HOWARD J. CLINEBELL

Fortress Press   Philadelphia

POCKET COUNSEL BOOKS

Am I Losing My Faith? by William E. Hulme
Drinking Problem? by John E. Keller
When Marriage Ends by Russell J. Becker
When Someone Dies by Edgar N. Jackson
The Middle Years by Paul E. Johnson
Crisis and Growth: Helping Your Troubled Child
    by Charlotte H. and Howard J. Clinebell

COPYRIGHT © 1971 BY FORTRESS PRESS

All rights reserved. No part of this publication may be reproduced, stored in a retrieval system, or transmitted in any form or by any means, electronic, mechanical, photocopying, recording, or otherwise, without the prior permission of the copyright owner.

Library of Congress Catalog Card Number 74-154490

ISBN 0-8006-1104-7

1672A71   Printed in the United States of America   1-1104

Series Introduction

Pocket Counsel Books are intended to help people with problems in a specific way. Problems may arise in connection with family life, marriage, grief, alcoholism, drugs or death. In addressing themselves to these and similar problems, the authors have made every effort to speak in language free from technical vocabulary.

Because these books are not only nontechnical but also brief, they offer a good start in helping people with specific problems. Face-to-face conversation between counselor and counselee is a necessary part of the help the authors envision through these books. The books are not a substitute for person-to-person counseling: they supplement counseling.

As the reader gets into a book dealing with his concerns, he will discover that the author aims at opening up areas of inquiry for further reflection. Thus through what is being read that which needs to be said and spoken out loud may come to the surface in dialog with the counselor. In "working through" a given problem in this personal way, help may come.

WILLIAM E. HULME
General Editor

As a Parent

—You care deeply about your children!
—You know more about them than anyone else does or will!
—Your basic hope and desire is for them to develop their full
   potential as creative persons!

A skilled professional may be able to help you use these vital resources more fully, but your love, understanding and hope are the most important elements in coping with problems and crises effectively.

Contents

1. ALL CHILDREN NEED HELP 1
   The Problems of Being a Parent, How to Make the Most of the Feeling Level, Parental Anger and the Setting of Limits

2. RECOGNIZING SERIOUS PROBLEMS 14
   Behavior Problems, Inner Disturbances, Psychosomatic Problems

3. UNDERSTANDING THE STAGES OF NORMAL DEVELOPMENT 24
   Infancy, Early Childhood, Play Age, School Age, Adolescence

4. FINDING HELP 34
   Sources of Reliable Information, What to Tell Your Child, What Will It Be Like, After Help

5. COPING WITH FAMILY CRISES 45
   Seven Guidelines, The Handicapped Child, Prolonged Illnesses, Drug Problems, One-Parent Families, Transmitting a Religious Orientation to Children

Preface

As a veteran beleaguered parent loaded with guilt and confusion, I decided to step back and try to figure out why, though many of the things I've read are partly helpful, I seem to harbor a sort of resentment toward all the authors of books for parents. I think it's because, while they all give lip service to the fact that parents are human beings, they then go on to expect superhuman behavior and emotional maturity from us.

We are to be firm but not rigid; flexible but not inconsistent; friendly but not palsy-walsy; provide wise, careful and constant guidance but encourage independence; set a good example of course; and never use threats, rewards or punishments. They all give the distinct impression that whatever is wrong with the child is the parents' (especially mother's) fault, and that's such a heavy burden to bear.

These heartfelt lines from a perceptive mother's letter express the intensity with which many parents feel the responsibility of raising children. Is it their fault when things go wrong with their children? Is their influence limited? Must they feel guilty and burdened? All human beings, including children, experience periods of unhappiness, stress, even downright misery. Most parents become concerned at times about whether their child is momentarily unhappy, passing through a stage, or facing a serious problem. They wonder whether to wait until it goes away, try to help their child themselves, or seek professional help.

As they grow, children encounter many large and small crises both expected and unexpected: birth itself, weaning, toilet training,

Preface

separation from parents, illness, accidents, the birth of a brother or sister, bad dreams, starting school, learning to read, making friends, adolescence—these and many other experiences provide the potential for problems of varying intensity. Most children cope with most of these experiences with reasonable success. But all children experience difficulty at certain points. Parents wonder, Will it go away? Can we help? Should we get professional help?

No family can avoid crises, either the normal everyday kind, or a sudden and unexpected blow. Serious illness or death in the family, job loss, financial worries, moving, new babies, marital conflict, children growing up and leaving home: these and many other experiences affect all family members profoundly. In the same family one child may be more adversely affected than another. Or a child may not appear to be affected at all. But parents wonder, How is my child taking this? Will it hurt him? How do we know? Does he need help, even if it doesn't show? Or, I know he is troubled. Should we get help for him? Where and how can we get it?

Increasingly, the overwhelming problems of the entire human family press upon us as individuals and families. The frightening seriousness of our destructive potential—nuclear war, a deteriorating environment, overpopulation—and the instant mass communication which keeps us constantly aware of the precariousness of human existence, make our anxieties high much of the time. Children are deeply affected both by these realities and by the anxiety they sense in their parents. So we ask ourselves, How can our children have a good life when everything is so uncertain? How can we help them become strong enough to cope with whatever they must face? Is there something special we can do to help our children be as happy and creative as is possible in an insecure, destructive world? Can our religious faith become a more vital force in our family relationships and in coping with crises?

The authors of this book know from personal as well as professional experience how heavily such questions can weigh on one's mind and marriage. As we share our experiences as family counselors, we hope that we will also communicate our empathy as

Preface

parents and as marriage partners. Worries about parent-child problems are painful. Each couple's pain is uniquely their own. But it helps to know that other parents feel similar pain and that people who try to counsel others have experiences of their own of the self-doubt, remorse, resentment, guilt, and fear, as well as the joy and fulfillment that accompany parent-child relationships.

Through our years of living, parenting, and counseling, we have acquired a deep respect for the strength and cope-ability of human beings. The remarkable resilience of people, including children, and the inner resources which they discover in the toughest circumstances, demonstrate this strength. Our hope is that what we say in these pages will help you as parents to appreciate your strengths and affirm your successes as well as to discover your unused inner resources. We hope that it will help to relieve the burden of guilt and confusion we all feel when things go wrong with our children.

Struggling to get the ideas in this book on paper has reminded us again and again of those persons who have taught us the most about parent-child relationships—our own parents and our three children. For their gifts of the past and of the future and for the myriad complexities of our relationships with them, we are profoundly grateful.

HOWARD and CHARLOTTE CLINEBELL

1.

All Children Need Help

The Problems of Being a Parent

Betsy won't give up the bottle. Will I have to let her go to kindergarten with it?

Tommy is just impossible! Everything he does is wrong and he does it on purpose! He's a bad boy!

Pete is always playing with matches. I'm afraid he's going to burn the house down.

Melinda didn't seem to care when her grandmother died. She didn't even cry. Now she hardly misses her. It doesn't seem right; she loved her grandmother so much.

Anita is so unhappy. She won't talk to me about it. What have I done wrong?

Alex fights all the time. He can't seem to get along well with the other boys at all.

Neal still wets the bed. His grandmother says he'll grow out of it. But it worries me.

Jack took some money out of my purse the other day. At this rate he'll become a juvenile delinquent!

Carla took too many pills the other night. I can't understand what she's got to worry so much about.

These statements of parents who were looking for help or were deciding whether to look for help reflect the bewilderment, hurt,

All Children Need Help

confusion and worry about their success as parents and the happiness of their child. It's hard to be a parent—maybe the hardest job there is. Most of us received almost no training for it. Nevertheless, we tend to be hard on ourselves. We expect of ourselves infinite wisdom, and understanding, unfailing patience, and above all, no mistakes. The remarkable and reassuring fact is that in spite of the difficult job and our lack of training for it most of us do a reasonably adequate job of parenting most of the time.

When things go wrong—and they do for everyone at times—we usually have one of three reactions: we fall into the guilt trap—blaming ourselves for our child's unhappiness; or we blame the child—he is bad, lazy or stupid; or we ignore the problem—pretending that it doesn't exist or hoping it will go away. These reactions are different ways of dealing with our anxieties about our success or failure as parents. None of them is usually helpful, either for ourselves or for our children.

Fourteen-year-old Anita spoke up in a group of young people who were discussing their problems and feelings. "I can't talk to my parents when I'm unhappy. They think it's all their fault. They feel so guilty that I feel guilty because I made them feel guilty." To which Nelia added, "They always want to make it better. They think you have to be happy all the time. They don't seem to know that you have to be miserable sometimes. I wish my mother would just cry with me instead of trying to make it all go away."

These girls are expressing what many children of all ages feel—the burden of having to feel happy all the time, so that their parents will not feel guilty. Our responsibility as parents is not to protect our children from all unhappiness but to help them to deal with it when, inevitably, it comes. The most helpful question is not "What did I do wrong?" but "What's the best way to help?" Sometimes the answer is simply to share our children's pain with them. Pain is an inevitable part of life. Much of the pain children experience is not the fault of parents. It is the price of being human.

Of course, being human we make mistakes in our relationships. Often it is well to admit our mistakes to our children. This helps

All Children Need Help

them to learn that it is human to be wrong sometimes, and a strength, not a weakness, to be able to admit it.

Sometimes we try to defend ourselves against our guilt and fear of failure by blaming the child.

Seven-year-old Tommy came for play therapy because he was misbehaving at home and at school. He fought with the boys, teased the girls, hurled obscenities at the teachers when they tried to control him. At home he broke his little sister's toys, hurt the baby, and refused to change no matter how frequently or brutally he was spanked. During his first play session as he moved destructively from the blocks to the dolls to the paint and clay, he turned momentarily to the therapist whom he had noticed was making notes. "What are you writing down? That I'm bad?"

Already at seven, Tommy had an inner picture of himself as a "bad boy." Parents, teachers, and other adults continually reinforced this image, verbally and physically, so that Tommy had to keep doing worse things to bring on worse punishments for the bad boy he felt himself to be. Of course we're not ignoring the fact that he had some responsibility for his "bad" behavior. Early in their lives, children must develop increasing and appropriate accountability for their behavior. But blaming the child and expecting him to do all the changing is as futile and destructive as taking all the blame ourselves.

The third way of dealing with our children's problems which tempts all of us at times is the "Maybe if I ignore it, it'll go away" method. And in fact, sometimes it does. But carried to the extreme, this way can be dangerous.[1]

Carla, fifteen, seemed depressed. Over a short period of time she had changed from a lively teen-ager to a withdrawn young person who began to avoid her friends, to drop out of activities, stay at home, shut herself in her room. At times she remarked that nothing seemed worthwhile any more. Once her father asked her what the matter was. She replied, "Oh, life just doesn't seem worth living." Her father laughed reassuringly. "Oh, Carla, at your age you don't have that many prob-

1. Some parents actually carry this method to the point of irresponsibility, not recognizing or admitting problems until someone outside the family—the school or the law—insists on it.

All Children Need Help

lems." Some time later she asked her mother how she would feel if she, Carla, committed suicide. Carla's mother laughed reassuringly. "Oh, Carla! You'll get over it." A few days later, Carla took an overdose of tranquilizers. Carla's cry for help was finally heard. Suddenly the doctor, the hospital, the police, her family all were hovering over her. Fortunately the pill bottle had been half empty. And her little brother had been there when it happened. Later, in family therapy, Carla's mother said, "I knew she was unhappy but I thought it was just a stage." Carla's father said, "I thought she just wanted us to feel sorry for her." Carla said, "I've been so miserable for so long, and nobody even cared."

Carla's parents didn't recognize her desperate distress signals. How do you know when your child's problems are serious and he needs more help than you can give? How do you avoid the guilt, blame, and head-in-sand traps? Is there any way of relating to children that will help them to be more secure and help parents not to feel like failures?

Whether your goal in reading this book is to increase your understanding of your children, to develop mutually satisfying parent-child intimacy, to gain insight or guidance in deciding whether your child needs professional help, the model we are suggesting can be summed up in these words, "Don't be afraid of feelings."

How to Make the Most of the Feeling Level

"When I talk about my feelings, I want my parents to be a long ways away."

Jason's family had come for help because of his severe learning problems at school. In the playroom the children were discovering a new level of relationship. Jason's statement followed the therapist's question, "How would it be to invite your mother and father to join us next week?" Through their work in the playroom Jason and his brother had learned that people love and hate each other at the same time. Jason had discovered and admitted to himself that he was jealous of his older brother's outstanding school record because he felt he could never measure up. The children had learned to play out their feelings with the puppets and to talk about them

All Children Need Help

freely. But so far the children did not feel that their newfound freedom with feelings could be used with their parents too. So the consensus was expressed by Jason, "No, I don't think they're ready for this sort of thing yet." (Actually they were. They too had been learning new ways of handling feelings in their own sessions. It took time for the children to believe their parents had changed too.)

It is not surprising that the feeling climate in many families is based on the rule, "feelings, especially negative feelings, are to be hidden." We were raised that way; so were our parents. We tend to pass on to our children the same limited range of permitted feeling. But there is a way of relating within families that can enhance the good times, make the bad times more bearable, and provide a way of anticipating and dealing with problems.

Psychiatrist Norman Paul[2] suggests that this way of relating begins with the development of "parental empathy"—the bond between a husband and wife which enables them to share with each other their fears, anxieties, despairs, joys and triumphs. Parental empathy is the ability of each parent to experience what the other feels—not should feel, but does feel! A husband and wife who struggle for a deeper level in their relationship can relate to their children at a deeper level.

When Betsy's mother expressed her anxiety about weaning, her husband's reply was, "But she's only a year old! She's not ready to give it up yet!" This interchange began a discussion about what was the appropriate age for a baby to give up the bottle. It lasted for several days, becoming increasingly heated. What began as a simple discussion over an apparently objective issue had mushroomed into a battle. He exclaimed angrily, "You're just like your mother, a hostile old witch, trying to take bottles away from babies!" She retorted, "Your mother is worse. She spoiled you rotten!"

Fortunately, Betsy's parents sought professional help, not so much to decide about weaning as to interrupt their own painful battles. How could a simple remark about a baby and her bottle

---

2. Norman Paul in *Parenthood: Its Psychology & Psychopathology,* ed. E. J. Anthony and T. Benedek (Boston: Little, Brown & Co., 1970), p. 16.

All Children Need Help

trigger a marital war? (Similar "objective" issues had triggered major fiascoes before.) They discovered in the course of counseling that the question of Betsy's bottle stirred up many feelings from the past still active in the present, as well as unfaced feelings in their current relationship. Betsy's mother discovered such feelings as, "Will I be a good mother if I let Betsy have the bottle any longer? What would my mother say if she heard Betsy still had the bottle after a year? Will Betsy stop loving me if I make her give up the bottle before she's ready?" Similarly her husband had mixed and unrecognized feelings in response to his wife's anxieties—his feelings of what a father and husband should be like, and his uncertainty about success in these roles, and the feelings toward his little daughter which stirred up his forgotten childhood feelings. As mother and father developed some awareness of their own and the other's deeper feelings and became more able to communicate about these feelings, mutual empathy began to develop. As parental empathy develops, external issues become easier to discuss rationally—is there a right age for weaning, what are the pros and cons, how important is it? When the feelings, positive and negative, which both partners bring to a problem are experienced openly and dealt with directly, they do not cloud and complicate the issue. Furthermore, "the issue" may seem much less important than before.

The rewarding by-product of this way of dealing with problems is increased husband-wife intimacy, which makes the marriage more satisfying and therefore makes them better parents.

Betsy's parents had no difficulty in acknowledging and expressing their anger toward each other. This ability to bring negative feeling out into the open can be an asset in a relationship. Facing and working through anger and conflict is the path to deeper intimacy. Healthy conflict clears the air, clarifies feelings, lets each person know where the other stands, and may lay the foundation for resolution of the problem. But when an argument continues for many days, increasing in heat or widening the gulf of cold resentment, it cannot lead to empathy, intimacy or the negotiation and resolution of differences.

All Children Need Help

Some couples take a different tack. Instead of a verbal confrontation when a misunderstanding appears likely, they withdraw, keeping all feelings to themselves in order to avoid conflict or pain. Melinda's parents (also quoted earlier) had perfected the "Don't let anybody, even yourself, know how you feel," method. For instance, early in their marriage Melinda's mother felt hurt and disappointment because sexual intercourse was often not satisfying. Because she felt she "shouldn't" feel that way, that it must be her fault, that her husband would be angry if he knew, she kept her feelings to herself. Her husband knew that things were not going as they should. But he felt that it was his fault, that he wasn't the man he thought he was, that his wife must think less of him, that he must try harder the next time. He, too, kept his feelings hidden. Neither dared share painful feelings with the other. Thus, each assumed feelings in the other that were not there. They also lost the opportunity to discover that the sexual relationship is a growing one, usually not fully satisfying at first. Because they could not share their own and experience each other's feelings, they withdrew little by little from each other. Each time one or the other was hurt in any area of their relationship, he stored up more anger which eventually became hidden not only from the other, but from himself. Their hidden, frozen feelings gradually blocked feelings of warmth, love, esteem and even sexual attraction.

Of course, Melinda quickly learned this way of handling her feelings. When she fell down and hurt herself someone always said, "Oh, it doesn't hurt. Don't cry!" When she felt angry at her new baby brother for getting so much attention, someone said, "Of course you love your little brother." When she started to school everyone said, "Don't be afraid. You'll like school." By adolescence Melinda was "programmed" to hide her feelings, even from herself. When grandmother died, she appeared not to care. For some reason, Melinda's mother was upset by her daughter's lack of feeling and sought help. Perhaps she sensed Melinda's loneliness and isolation. Perhaps she was simply tired of her own. The family was soon involved in family therapy, where gradually they learned to

All Children Need Help

share the gift of their feelings, to tell each other when they were angry or disappointed or hurt. They also began to be able to tell each other when they were glad, or felt good about each other. As Melinda said after many weeks of family therapy, "You know it isn't just that I was never sad. I was never glad either. I just put all my feelings away in a box. But now, when I cry because grandmother died and I miss her, I also remember how she used to sing to me. And that feels good. Isn't it strange that you can be glad and sad at the same time and you can't have either one without the other?"

This bit of wisdom from a fourteen-year-old girl who was discovering her feelings describes the reality of being human. We live fully only if we allow ourselves to experience the full range of feeling. We are free to feel deeply joyful and loving only if we are also free to feel pain and anger and despair.

Betsy's and Melinda's families utilized professional help to discover feelings and unravel problems. They moved on to fuller marital and parent-child intimacy following help. Professional help is by no means always so successful; nor is it always necessary. Parents are often able to develop empathy between themselves and with their children on their own. (The books listed at the end of this chapter provide guidelines for people who want to make the most of the feeling level in their marriage or family.)

Max comes home from the fourth grade class one day feeling angry and discouraged. "Oh, I have so much homework! That teacher makes us work too hard." Max's father says, "Oh now, Max, you can't learn anything if you don't do your homework. The teacher is showing you that you have to work hard in this world." Well, all that may be true, and no doubt Max knows it already. Probably he hadn't really questioned the fact that the homework had to be done. But Max feels, "My father doesn't understand. It's no use telling him how I feel." A consistent diet of nonunderstanding forces feelings underground. Sooner or later, Max lashes out with some form of misbehavior at school, or he does a poor job with his school work, or he becomes compulsive about his work to

All Children Need Help

try to meet his parents' expectations; he may grow up driving himself to the sort of "success" which will keep him from discovering the deep satisfactions of human relationships or make him more vulnerable to ulcers and heart attacks.

But suppose Max's father had said,

F : "Feeling pretty discouraged about having to work some more when the school day is over, eh Max?"

M: "Boy, and how! I really don't want to do my homework at all!"

F : "You feel like just forgetting it all?"

M: "Yeah! But I guess I'll get it over with so I can watch TV tonight. . . ."

What Max feels is, "Boy, my dad really knows what it's like to feel this way." That's empathy! No parent can be empathetic all the time. But a family which communicates empathetically much of the time prevents many problems from arising or from becoming unmanageable. (Of course, unless this way of accepting negative feelings has become a pattern, the story won't end so happily. And even if it is a pattern there are times when parents simply have to insist on the behavior they expect from a child whether he likes it or not.

A pattern of family empathy helps prevent problems from getting out of hand by cultivating a climate in which family members feel free to share their inner fears and disappointments. Recall Carla's story. When Carla said, "Life doesn't seem worth living any more," her father and mother responded with, "Oh, Carla, you don't have that many problems" and "You'll get over it." But what Carla heard inside herself was, "They don't understand. They don't think it's important. They don't know how I feel." She withdrew into her own world of misery. If either parent had been able to say something like, "You're feeling pretty low about things these days," the door might have been opened for Carla to talk about her troubles; the withdrawal, the loneliness, the suicide attempt might have been prevented. Sharing, recognizing, and experiencing feellings in the here and now often keeps them from causing trouble in the future.

All Children Need Help

Parental Anger and the Setting of Limits

You may have the impression that we've been saying that parents must always be calm, understanding, patient, and wise. This is definitely not what we believe. Even if it were possible (which it isn't) it wouldn't be desirable. Children need to learn from parental example how to handle negative feelings. Parents are people, too! We also feel confusion, anger, pain, frustration, hurt, disappointment and resentment as well as joy, passion and love. And we have the same need to own and express these feelings. Parents who can argue vehemently, resolve the differences in some way, and become friends again, are showing their children that anger is an acceptable, often useful emotion. They are teaching their children how to use it constructively. Parents who can grieve deeply when there is a sadness of some kind are teaching their children that pain is an important part of being human and needs to be recognized and felt.

How we express anger towards our children is vitally important. Haim Ginott[3] suggests a direct statement of the parent's feeling rather than an attack on the child's character. Instead of "Oh, you bad boy. How could you be so stupid?" a mother could say, "It makes me furious when you track mud onto my clean rug!" In the first instance, the child feels inside, "I'm bad. I'm stupid." In the second he thinks, "Wow, it sure makes mother mad when I get mud on her carpet!" Ordinarily children don't want to incur their parent's wrath—at least not consistently (unless that is their only way of getting noticed).

This leads to setting limits. A family cannot be a full democracy. Children should participate in family decisions when it is appropriate but parents must retain the veto power in important matters. Children need to know where the limits are. Matthew, two, runs into the street. His mother brings him back instantly and makes it clear he must not do this again. Here is a firm limit he must accept whether he understands or not. Of course his mother also can expect his fury at being thus controlled. For a two-year-old, a brief explosion of temper would be a normal response.

3. Haim Ginott, *Between Parent and Child* (New York: Avon Books, 1965).

All Children Need Help

By the time Matthew is ten, things are different. The rules (limits) are different. He has more freedom according to his growing ability to be responsible for his own safety. Parental discipline is different. It's important that he understand and accept the limits, even if he doesn't like them. But feelings are as important as ever. Matthew now understands and respects the street. He knows how far and under what circumstances he can go on his bike. But one day he goes too far and comes home late. Matt's father is worried and angry and he shows it! He says Matt may not ride his bike at all tomorrow. Matt is furious. He had planned to ride to the park with his friend tomorrow. Instead of a two-year-old temper tantrum he says angrily to his father, "I hate you!" Matt's father recalls his own childhood and how mad he used to get at his father. He knows how it feels from both the child's and the parent's side. He replies, "I know you're angry. I was mad too when you broke the rule. I was worried about you. I know you wanted to go to the park tomorrow. But you will have to manage without your bike." Matt turns angrily away. On his way through the garage to the house he pounds furiously at the punching bag for several minutes. (Matt's father, on his way in, hits the punching bag hard a few times himself!)

This family has rules. Matt is expected to adhere to them even though they don't always seem reasonable to him. This family experiences conflict. Close relationships and conflict always go together. This family respects feelings. Matt was angry because of the punishment. His father recognized and accepted Matt's anger without allowing it to control his handling of the situation. Matt's father was also free to express his own anger. Matt knows by now there is no use arguing with his father; he'll just have to get to the park some other way, or else stay home. But he can accept the punishment more easily because he knows his feelings are also accepted, even though he doesn't get over his anger right away.

As it becomes a family pattern, this way of setting limits and handling anger pays off in less frequent conflict, more constructive handling of it when it does arise, and in increasing respect for necessary authority. In contrast recall Tommy's family. At seven

All Children Need Help

Tommy already saw himself as bad and behaved accordingly. Tommy's parents could not tolerate anger directly expressed by their son. When he misbehaved, they called him a bad boy but they neither listened to his feelings nor let him know ahead of time what the limits were and what consequences would follow.

Sometimes parents succeed in coercing their children into obedience through too rigid limits and punishment without dealing with the inevitable feelings involved. Sooner or later, these feelings make themselves known—in destructive ways; sometimes not until those children become parents themselves.

Freedom of feeling does not mean freedom of destructive action. It is appropriate for Matt to express his anger verbally to his father and to pound the punching bag. It would not be appropriate for him to strike his father. Children should never be allowed to hit parents since this makes them feel very guilty and teaches them a destructive pattern for expressing anger. Children want and need to learn, through the firm setting of limits, that their angry, destructive impulses can be controlled. A child who learns from the beginning that his strong feelings are healthy and legitimate and that there are appropriate ways of expressing them gradually develops inner controls. He grows up with an inner respect for authority—his own as well as others. He develops self-control because he has experienced discipline as an expression of caring in a relationship of love.

Some parents are too permissive. They do not provide their children with the security of knowing how far they can go. Destructive acting out behavior by these children is usually a cry for help: "Please, somebody, stop me. Help me learn how to stop myself."

Other parents are too authoritarian. They set too many unreasonable rules, punish too severely, and refuse to allow questioning of limits or expression of anger. Their children become compliant, frightened and submissive or burst out violently with destructive actions.

But between these two extremes is rational authority. Parents who use this means set limits where they are necessary and make them appropriate to the child's age, and encourage and accept the ex-

All Children Need Help

pression of the child's feeling. As they grow older these children gradually take more and more responsibility for setting their own limits until they, like their parents, become responsible adults.

Although this is the ideal, we are all human, and we often fall short of our own goals. Even when we understand the importance of feelings, and make the effort to deal with them honestly, we often fail. There are outside forces—influences of school, community, the wide, wide world. Since most of us were not raised to deal with feelings openly, we miss many opportunities to meet each other empathetically. Also, most of us adults experienced at least one painful stage in our early lives from which we still carry unhealed wounds or sensitive scars; when our children hit that stage, we feel anxious and inadequate. Some of us are great with babies and inept with teen-agers or vice versa.

It is comforting to realize that if the overall feeling tone and emotional climate of the family is positive we can make many mistakes without permanent damage to our children.

Still, there are times when things go wrong and we need outside help. Chapter Two will discuss how we can recognize those times.

Recommended Reading

Axline, Virginia M., *Dibs: In Search of Self* (Boston: Houghton Mifflin Co., 1965). How play therapy helped a little boy and his family.

Baruch, Dorothy W., *New Ways in Discipline, You and Your Child Today* (New York: McGraw-Hill Book Co., 1949). Dealing with children's feelings.

Ginott, Haim G., *Between Parent and Child* (New York: Avon Books, 1965) and *Between Parent and Teenager* (New York: Macmillan Co., 1969). Practical suggestions about parent-child and parent-teen communication.

Harris, Thomas, *I'm OK, You're OK* (New York: Harper & Row, 1969).

2.

Recognizing Serious Problems

"There is no single piece of behavior, no matter how unusual it seems, that may not be, at one time or other, in the behavioral repertoire of every child."[1]

Nearly everyone can profit from competent help at times. But the question of when it would be merely helpful and when it is essential is a major one. When you suspect that a problem has developed or is developing, there are a number of questions you should ask which will help you decide whether or not to get outside help.

Question One. Is the particular behavior you are worried about age appropriate—that is, can it be considered normal for a child of this particular age? Neal's parents were worried about his bedwetting. The counselor with whom they talked asked his age. Neal was three years old. The counselor explained that while many little boys have stopped wetting the bed at three, many have not. If the parents can relax and be patient, probably Neal's bed-wetting will stop of its own accord. If the bed-wetting is continuing when Neal is four or five they may want to raise the question again. By this time much depends on whether the issue has become a battleground within the family.

Betsy and the bottle provide another example. Drinking from a bottle can certainly be considered normal behavior for an eighteen-month-old child. The main issue was how her parents felt about it.

---

1. Howard M. Halpern, *A Parent's Guide to Child Psychotherapy* (New York: A. S. Barnes and Co., 1963), p. 36.

Recognizing Serious Problems

But a child who is still demanding a bottle regularly when he starts to school, probably needs help with deeper problems. Of course, many young children, right up through elementary school, want to "regress" (play at being a baby again) sometimes. When a new baby comes or growing-up pressures become intense, all children feel like retreating temporarily. It is well to recognize this need verbally and go along with it. An older child allowed to lie down on the floor with the bottle while his baby sister is being fed, will soon leave the need behind if he has his parents' tolerant acceptance. If he doesn't leave it behind, a deeper problem which does need help is there. Allowing the child to try out the bottle again does not cause the problem. (It may give parents a chance to discover if one is there.)

Jack was ten years old when his mother found him taking money out of her purse. It developed that he was also taking things from others at school, and once in a while from a store. Jack's parents did well to seek help. At ten years old, Jack knew better. His behavior was a symptom of deeper disturbance; his taking something his parents would be sure to discover was a cry for help. On the other hand, a three-year-old who takes money from mother's purse is usually behaving normally for a three-year-old. Mother merely needs to keep her purse put away.

There are times, of course, when behavior is dangerous, even when it is normal for a particular age. Pete was three when his father got upset over his playing with matches. But three-year-olds are fascinated with fire and not convinced of its danger. If he discovers matches within his reach he is likely to experiment with them. But if Pete were five or six or seven, or older, chronic fire play would indicate that help probably should be sought without delay. With all real or suspected problems in children the relation of age to the behavior is a crucial one.

Question Two. How severe is the problem? The issue of severity includes duration and frequency. How long has the problem been going on? How often does it happen? Is it getting more or less frequent?

Recognizing Serious Problems

Suppose Neal is still wetting the bed at five. Now his parents will ask themselves different questions. Did it stop for a while and begin again when the baby was born or Neal started to school? Does it happen only sometimes when Neal is under particular stress? If the answers are yes, the parents would do well to relax a while longer. Bed-wetting frequently returns temporarily when children are under pressure, even up to adolescence. Is the bed-wetting, though never completely stopped, getting less frequent of its own accord? Again, the parents should relax and be patient. Is the bed-wetting unabated or is it getting worse? Is it an important issue between Neal and his parents? If these two questions are answered "yes," then Neal's parents should check out the problem with a professional.

How about Jack taking money from mother's purse? We have decided that this is not acceptable behavior for a ten-year-old. But before we decide that Jack is a juvenile delinquent or even that his problem is severe enough to need professional help, we need to ask more questions. Is this an isolated incident or has it happened before? How often or under what circumstances? Is Jack angry because his parents refused him something he especially wanted to buy? Is he needing some money desperately for something he knows his parents would disapprove of, but which he feels he must have to keep up his image with his peers? All of us adults, if we allow ourselves to remember our childhoods, can recall times when we did things we shouldn't have done. It didn't mean we were on the road to crime, or moral depravity; it simply meant that we were often tempted and sometimes gave in. All children are like that. (How we respond to this human characteristic in our children helps to determine whether it has lasting negative effects.)

Sometimes mild problems which are normal at a particular age develop into severe symptoms that make getting help vital. Think again of Carla. Her feelings of despair and depression were not unusual for her age. Adolescence is a trying time for all young people; they experience a great deal of self-doubt, insecurity and fear as they wrestle with the physical and emotional changes which accompany growing up. But in Carla's case the symptoms were too

Recognizing Serious Problems

constant over too long a period of time and became increasingly severe. Prolonged depression, increasing withdrawal, or talk of death and suicide, always indicate a severe problem which needs immediate help.

The question of severity can be asked in practical terms—to what extent does a problem interfere with our child's normal living and relationships? Occasional insomnia may be a bothersome symptom of fears at a particular stage but if it keeps a young teen-ager from being able to attend slumber parties, it may be interfering with important learning experiences with peers or it may be the symptom of a deeper problem.

Question Three. Does the behavior you are concerned about represent an obvious personality change? Did it appear suddenly or for no apparent reason? In Carla's case there was a definite personality change in a fairly short period. A vivacious, outgoing, and active adolescent had become consistently depressed and withdrawn. Her parents commented frequently, "It isn't like Carla." Whenever that statement can be made unequivocally over a period of time, it is likely that help is needed. All of us have our ups and downs. But the ups and downs fit into our basic personality pattern. When "it just doesn't fit," then it may be that a child with a deeper disturbance is calling for help.

Alex's father was upset because his son fought all the time. "He didn't used to be like that at all. He got along fine in school last year. He's always had lots of friends. Everyone used to like him. But now he picks a fight with anyone who comes near him. The teacher at school says she can't even let him on the playground anymore." Although a certain amount of fighting is normal for school age boys, Alex's problem sounds severe and reflects a definite change in his personality. Alex needs help.

Even when the problem is not severe and can be considered normal for the age, any sudden or obvious change in personality should be watched. When in doubt, talk it over with a competent professional person.

Question Four. Is the child's behavior a reflection of other painful problems within the family? This is the hardest of the four ques-

Recognizing Serious Problems

tions. Parents often wonder why a counselor suggests that they themselves get help when it is obvious that the child has the problems. In any family, when one person is upset, all are upset. If the marriage is under stress, the family is under stress. If the children are upset, the marriage is put under additional pressure. A family is like an intricately spun web. When the entire web is disturbed, one strand may vibrate violently. A disturbed child is usually vibrating with the pain of the entire family network. He reflects pain in family relationships but his problem also increases the family pain.

Since the quality of the marriage sets the feeling tone for the family, parents should look at their own relationship when they are considering whether something is wrong with their child. Betsy's parents discovered this when they began to argue about the question of weaning. It was not so much Betsy's problem as theirs. At the same time, it created an opportunity for them to improve their marriage, for their sakes and for Betsy's. They dealt with their own problems in a marriage counseling relationship with their pastor. For Betsy it was fortunate that her parents had the courage and strength to get help early in her life. She might otherwise have increasingly become the focus of their battles. Couples often fight over a child in order to avoid facing the real issues between themselves. This is destructive to the child as well as to the marriage.

It is surprising how often what appears to be the child's problem turns out to be merely the symptom of an unhappy marriage. Alex's parents sought help for him because of the unhappiness evident in his inability to get along with other children. But the clinic where they took Alex also worked with his parents. There they were able to talk of their own problems—the fact that their marriage had been unhappy for some time, that they talked of divorce but felt they should stay together "for the children's sake." Although they had not talked directly with the children about it, Alex had sensed his parents' unhappiness. He didn't know why, but he felt frightened and angry. When he was asked why he got in so much trouble his reply was, "I don't know." And he didn't.

In play therapy sessions, his feelings began to come clear, even to himself. As he played with the doll family one day he described

Recognizing Serious Problems

aloud what was happening. "The father learns to fly. He flies right out of the house. The boy can't fly like the father can." Suddenly Alex stopped, a look of surprise and fear on his face. He turned to the therapist: "Sometimes I think my father will go away and I'll never see him again."

T.: "Things have been sort of unhappy at your house and you're afraid you might lose your father."

A.: "Yeah, my parents might get a divorce!"

No wonder Alex fought all the time. By keeping his parents' attention on himself, he may also have felt that he was "keeping them together." Getting the worry out in the open where it could be seen and understood was a great relief to Alex. In the meantime his parents had made some progress in working out their problems. Family sessions were arranged where parents and children could talk out their fears and angers with the help of a neutral person who could help them communicate effectively. When the parents could say, "Yes, we have some serious differences, but we're working on them," the children could also begin coping with their feelings. In this case both the marriage counseling and the play sessions for the children were continued for a while, with occasional meetings together, until the family felt they could continue the new communication patterns at home on their own. A blocked family had learned how to grow; mutual need satisfaction was replacing mutual starvation.

Of course it doesn't always work out so happily. Alex's parents might have decided that their differences were too great, that a divorce was the best course. Then it would be important for Alex and the other children (and adults) in the family to have help in dealing constructively with their feelings about that.

It is always possible that parents themselves can help their children in this way if they are skillful in dealing with their own feelings. If they have trouble with this, professional help is essential in order for family members to learn the communication skills they need to help themselves.

In the past, professional counselors assumed that a person with a problem needed to have one-to-one counseling or therapy. Most

Recognizing Serious Problems

child guidance clinics have been organized on this basis—the child had a problem; maybe the mother needed help in learning how to handle the child, but it was essentially the child who needed to be changed. That attitude has altered dramatically within the last few years. Nowadays, many professional counselors believe that when one family member is in pain, all family members are also suffering and need help. Abnormal symptoms in one member may be the result of his expressing the pain or acting out the hidden feelings in the whole family. This was true of Alex. Often it is true that the individual himself needs help—but he can change more easily (and stay changed) if the family pattern which to some degree causes and continues his problem is dealt with, too.

It is by no means always the case that a child's problems reflect obvious or overt marital conflicts. Empty marriages with little depth relationship and those engaged in a quiet "cold war" also produce disturbed children. But the children of relatively healthy marriages also have problems. There are powerful outside influences. Disturbing things happen at school. There is television. There are anxieties about war and nuclear holocaust and poisoned air. One television newscast can stir up tremendous anxiety even in adults. Children tend to sense these anxieties and internalize them. For young people there are the problems of peer relationships and the anxieties and risks involved in changing sexual standards. A family which communicates freely often becomes aware of potential problems (inside or outside the family) before they get out of hand. But not always. And no parents are always fully sensitive to each other and their children. (The tendency of some parents, of course, is to blame "outside bad influence" and ignore the problems within their marriage which are disturbing the child.)

Types of Problems

Specialists in child therapy often separate childhood problems into (1) those which are expressed outwardly in troubled and troubling behavior, (2) those which are experienced inwardly as troubled, conflicted feelings such as extreme fears or shyness, and

Recognizing Serious Problems

(3) those in which tensions and conflicts interfere with the functioning of some system of the child's body producing psychosomatic problems. These are not clear-cut or exclusive categories; a child may combine all three—behavior difficulties, neurotic problems, and psychosomatic symptoms. Recognizing some of these symptoms early often prevents more serious problems in the future.

Behavior Problems

The majority of parents who seek help for a child do so because the child's outward behavior worries them or someone outside the family, often the school authorities or law enforcement officers. Here are some frequent behavior problems:

Aggressive and destructive behavior: almost all children are aggressive and destructive at times but children who constantly pick fights with other children, hurt themselves or others, or consistently disrupt the classroom in defiance of authority, need help. When strenuous efforts by both parents and teacher prove ineffective it is essential to get the help of a specialist in child or family therapy.

Lying and stealing: the age of the child and the frequency and severity of the behavior determine when these symptoms point to the need for help. All children tell untruths at times, often to protect themselves from punishment; some children have spells of telling wild stories which are simply fantasies; many children sometimes take something they shouldn't. But persistent lying and stealing at any age is a cry for help; professional counseling should be obtained.

Excessive preoccupation with sex: all children are interested in their own and each others' bodies; all children are interested in what goes on in their parents' bedroom. All children experiment sometimes. People are fascinated by sex at any age. But if free and open communication about it or relaxed handling of normal but inappropriate behavior does not suffice, then help is needed. Masturbation is normal at any age. But if it is excessive or produces guilt or interferes with a child's normal activities, it is symptomatic of a deeper unhappiness.

Recognizing Serious Problems

Learning problems are sometimes called inadequate functioning rather than behavior problems. They may stem from unrealistic adult expectations, from inadequate intellectual stimulation or from emotional conflicts. If extra tutoring and a relaxed attitude do not change the situation, help should be sought.

Inner Disturbances

Children who are disturbed or unhappy do not always act in ways that upset adults. Quiet, shy children are sometimes simply that—there's nothing wrong with being quiet or shy. But if this quietness is excessive, it may mean there are problems.

Inadequate relationships are involved in all the problems we have discussed. But this may be the primary focus of the problem if the child is unable to establish close relationships with either adults or peers. People are different. Some need many friends. Some need a few. But all of us need someone. A child who is a "loner" or who is happy only with adults needs help.

Extreme withdrawal is a symptom of deep disturbance. A child who does not seem interested in anyone, who stays alone too much, or who suddenly withdraws when he has always been outgoing is in need of help.

Extreme fears always indicate need for help of some kind. Often parents can help their children simply by listening, understanding and reassuring. But when the fears consistently interfere with normal activities—sleeping, going to school, doing the things required by the child's particular life stage, accomplishing the things he wants to accomplish—then help should be sought. School phobia, the child's refusing to go to school, is an example of extreme fear which interferes with functioning; parents should seek help at once.

Speech problems vary in seriousness. Many, sometimes even stuttering, are passing problems. But if they go on too long and interfere with the child's functioning or relationships he needs help.

Bizarre behavior should never be ignored. It may indicate the onset of severe mental disturbance. A child who acts inappropriately to the objective circumstance, who deliberately injures himself without complaint, or engages in repetitious motions such as head-banging or rocking should have help at once.

Psychosomatic Problems

Children often express their conflicts in living through their bodies. Asthma, rashes, hay fever, colitis, frequent colds, stomach aches, headaches, and other ailments may have their roots in emotional conflicts as well as physiological weaknesses in that particular organ system. Children frequently develop physical symptoms when they have big feelings which they cannot express openly (and of which they may not be consciously aware).

It is important to check out all physical symptoms with a pediatrician or family doctor. If no physical basis is discovered for the problem, and it persists, the services of a child therapist or a family therapist may be what is needed. Emotions have a powerful effect on the body and the realm of emotions is the realm of relationships —the improvement of which is the goal of counseling. It is important, of course, to have regular medical checkups—even if a child's problems don't express themselves physically. Sometimes medical problems are hidden behind behavior and personality problems. Sometimes, also, a doctor can help to decide whether the problem needs attention or is simply a stage of normal development.

Recommended Reading

Chess, Stella et al., *Your Child Is a Person* (New York: Viking Press, 1965). Understanding your child's individuality.

Gruenberg, Sidonie M., *The Parents' Guide to Everyday Problems of Boys and Girls* (New York: Random House, 1959). Covers ages 5 to 12.

3.

Understanding the Stages of Normal Development

> When we think of all the things that seemed like king-sized problems at the time but turned out to be just a part of Jimmy's particular stage, it helps us keep some perspective on our current collection of parental worries.

This statement by a father in a parents' growth group is probably true to the experience of most families. The vast majority of child problems turn out to be temporary upsets or passing phases. Some parents, though, go into an emotional tailspin about normal developmental problems. By "making a federal case" out of what would ordinarily pass as the child matures, they may actually prevent the problem from passing. The child may remain stuck in negative behavior or attitudes because he has discovered that they get him giant helpings of parental concern and attention. On the other hand, what appears to be a passing problem may actually be the onset of a major difficulty from which the child won't recover without professional help. An understanding of the kinds of stresses, crises, and difficulties that are "par for the course" for children at successive growth stages in our culture, can help quiet unnecessary parental anxieties and, at the same time, alert you to real distress signals. Knowledge of normal development can provide general guidelines in deciding what is "age appropriate" and when to seek profes-

Understanding the Stages of Normal Development

sional help. Knowing about normal development is also valuable in your efforts to facilitate your child's maturing—a positive approach to preventing problems.

Problems and growing up go together. At each new life stage, a person must learn new, untried ways of relating so as to get his basic needs for love, acceptance, understanding, freedom, and achievement satisfied. This is a risky, threatening task, yet the growth drive that is in everyone also creates a strong desire to move ahead. This is the conflict—whether to stay where you are comfortable and secure, or to risk moving to the next stage. Each life stage has its central task. Serious problems occur when a person doesn't accomplish the life assignment of his developmental stage. When he moves on chronologically without the inner security of knowing that tasks at the previous stages were relatively well completed, the new stage is more threatening and difficult. It's like constructing a building without a sturdy foundation. Thus, serious problems stem from blocked growth. Conversely, to the extent that a person fulfills his personality potential, serious problems are prevented. A person who is moving toward the fulfillment of his unique potentialities as an individual, will have problems (like the rest of the human race), but he will be able to handle them and even use them as an opportunity for further growth.

Each person has his own unique growth pattern. Each child matures according to his individual pattern. Anxious parents who unwittingly put pressure on a child to conform to what's "normal" for his age group forget that such norms are only statistical averages of a wide, wide range of individual differences. Respect for a child's own inner developmental pattern and timetable is an indispensable ingredient in parent-child acceptance. Each family also changes in its own unique way, as parents and children together evolve that family's "personality," its style of relationship and pattern of development.

Let us now look more closely at the developmental tasks, pressures, and problems which are typical of the five childhood-youth stages,[1]

---

1. We are using the first five of Erik Erikson's "Eight Stages of Man," in *Childhood and Society,* 2nd ed. (New York: W. W. Norton and Co., 1963).

Understanding the Stages of Normal Development

remembering that these aren't developmental boxes but broad generalizations about each life stage.

Stage One: INFANCY (Birth to 15 months). The life task of this stage is developing basic trust, the deep dependable conviction that "life is okay and I'm okay."[2] Basic trust (or basic mistrust) grows within the parent-infant relationship. A baby with a solid, loving tie with a mothering person, who in turn has a trustful nurturing marriage, will acquire a deep conviction that life and relationships can be trusted to satisfy his basic needs. Erik Erikson, who has explored the life stages most extensively, calls this "basic faith in existence." Basic trust is the foundation of identity and self-trust, enabling one to form trustful relationships throughout life—in marriage, with children, with society, with God.

The details of child-rearing practices aren't really the important thing. The quality of the nurturing relationship is important! Parents who take pleasure in nurturing—feeding, cuddling, rocking, cooing to the baby—communicate to him empathetically the deep sense of being okay. The father who is comfortable in his masculinity can enjoy sharing with mother the tender, nurturing of the baby. Security comes to a baby via body love, including abundant sucking and warm body contact with the nurturing ones. The contemporary companionship model of marriage—a relationship of genuine intimacy that is possible only between true equals—frees both partners to enjoy the co-nurturing of the new life they have created together. The concept of responsible family planning means that parents will only have children who are wanted and who can be well nurtured by them.

Many later problems of children are rooted in inadequacies in this first, trust-forming stage—depression, feelings of unworth, withdrawal from relationships, continued infantile behavior such as thumbsucking and overeating, for example. Some adult problems also have their roots in stage one—alcoholism, schizophrenia, manic-depressive mood swings, excessive smoking, criticizing, and suspiciousness. The experiences of stage one lay the foundation for later

2. Thomas Harris, *I'm OK, You're OK* (New York: Harper & Row, 1969).

Understanding the Stages of Normal Development

religious trust. A child's most important lessons in theology are learned before his first birthday as he acquires the deep conviction that existence is or is not trustworthy.

Stage Two: EARLY CHILDHOOD (15 months to 2½ years). The main growth task of a child at this stage is to develop a sense of selfhood (autonomy) as a separate person. A child's intense wish to choose and his vigorous "No" saying around age two show that his sense of self is emerging, being tested and strengthened in opposition to the wills around him. Feelings about his body and about the demands of society grow strong as he is confronted with the expectation that he become toilet trained. This is an early and therefore a decisive confrontation with the demands of society and the self-discipline required to live together in a social group. The controls by his parents need to be firmly reassuring to protect him from the potential anarchy of his untrained inner urges. Lack of limits and discipline will be experienced as rejection. If discipline is both loving and firm, he will begin to conform without the loss of basic trust and self-esteem. But, if discipline is heavy-handed, arbitrary, unpredictable, or divorced from love, then shame and self-doubt result.

Children who are afraid of dirt and too neat, compulsively organized in every area of life, obsessed by feelings that the body is unclean, or who mess everything they touch, are experiencing problems rooted at the early childhood stage. The issue here is the balance between freedom and control. Children who feel a sense of "self-control without loss of self-esteem" are able to combine good feelings of autonomy and cooperation with others. Parents who have a relatively comfortable feeling about their own bodies and a firm sense of autonomy transmit these affirming feelings to their children during this stage.

Stage Three: PLAY AGE (2½ to 6). The development of a sturdy sense of self continues as the child becomes aware not just that he is a person (autonomy), but what kind of person. The key life task of this stage is developing initiative—being able to move about aggressively, try out and like the thrust of his personality. Increasing language and muscular abilities give him a good inner sense

Understanding the Stages of Normal Development

of mastery. Consuming curiosity is a sign that he is moving out aggressively with his mind to grasp and understand his world.

Sibling rivalry often is intense during this period (perhaps earlier). Preoccupation with sexual differences (discovered in this or the preceding period) is strong. Normally a child's feelings of his own sexual identity are awakened during this time by a warm relationship with the parent of the opposite sex. Fantasies, often frightening to the child, of taking the place of the same-sexed parent are present. The child's need is for a dependable, loving relationship with both parents, and for them to have a strong relationship with each other so that he will know that eventually he must move beyond this way of satisfying his needs.

Having been awakened to the wonderful awareness of his sexuality during this period, a child lets go of his fantasies and his close attachment to the opposite-sexed parent. He resolves the oedipal dilemma (of wanting to have an exclusive relationship with the opposite-sexed parent but recognizing that he or she is already "taken") by identifying with the same-sexed parent in the next stage. However, if the boy's father (or the girl's mother) isn't available (emotionally or physically) the child may become trapped (fixated) in the oedipal attachment. If the opposite-sexed parent is too dependent on the child for emotional satisfactions because of the lack of a satisfying marriage or other adult relationship, the same fixation may occur. When one is stuck in any life stage, blocked growth produces personality and relationship problems. Fixation in the oedipal stage may, for example, result in a "Mama's boy" or in neurotic anxieties about sex and fear of closeness to either sex.

Stage Four: SCHOOL AGE (6 to puberty). The child's key growth task during this stage is to achieve a sense of "industry"—derived from beginning to acquire the skills which will be useful to him as a man or woman. School experiences of success are important here, since they give a child a sense of budding competence in language, math, and thinking skills which are essential to subsequent school success and to adequate adult functioning. This is

Understanding the Stages of Normal Development

also the time when a girl absorbs female roles and a boy absorbs male ones.

But in our day definitions of masculine and feminine roles are changing dramatically. Many parents therefore are unsure about what is really appropriate for men and women. During the present transition period and until new definitions of maleness and femaleness emerge (probably allowing for much greater variety in roles among different couples) there is bound to be some confusion for the developing boy and girl. Although past roles were too rigid and constricting, they were more secure and easier to fit into than the present changing and often confused roles.[3]

Meanwhile, the importance of both male and female adults as models for normal development during this stage cannot be overemphasized. The old way of limiting mothers to home, and fathers to the outside world has often meant that children became too emotionally attached to mothers and too emotionally distant from fathers. Clinging mothers do not free their children to grow. Absentee fathers also have an adverse effect on sons and daughters. A girl in early adolescence, says family life educator Kay Crowe, needs a father who "makes her feel she is a budding woman with great possibilities for the future." If the father is emotionally or physically missing, the child usually picks up the mother's anger toward him (and men generally), because of her own unmet needs. Sons feel fatherly deprivation acutely during the oedipal periods and the school years (6–12), during which they are searching for a strong sense of their own maleness. Although the changes in male/female roles represented by the women's liberation movement will undoubtedly cause severe problems in some marriages, and therefore disturb the children, the eventual benefits for marriage, families and parent-child relationships are great.

3. Girls need no longer be programmed solely as future wives and mothers. Boys need no longer be expected to become sole providers, protectors and defenders of their women and children. The rapidly developing equality of the sexes opens a whole new world of sharing and developing their own pattern of male/female roles. It also means many more possibilities of creative development for both sexes, especially for women. The revolutionary change in roles is long overdue and potentially revitalizing to our society.

Understanding the Stages of Normal Development

During the second half of the school age stage, the child normally forms strong relationships with his own sex and age group; this is the so-called gang stage. Peer relationships and the wider society of adults outside the family (teachers, ministers, coaches) become increasingly important as sources of need satisfaction.

Achievement of a firm sense of "industry" (skill mastery) during this stage of learning helps a child enter subsequent stages without nagging feelings of inadequacy. Early school failure may cause the child to feel trapped in a failure cycle—in which each failure increases the probability of another failure. Children who learn to relate with peers in mutually satisfying ways, move into adolescence with feelings of adequacy within relationships.

Stage Five: ADOLESCENCE (Puberty to 20). The crucial life task of adolescence is to complete the sense of identity. Who am I? What am I worth? What can I do that is important? This is the pay-off period, when the successes and failures of previous stages make the adolescent's task much more or much less difficult. It is also a second-chance stage, when partially unfinished developmental tasks may be completed as a foundation for the life tasks of the three adult stages—intimacy (emotional and sexual) in young adulthood, generativity (being a generator or creator) in the middle years, and ego integrity (making peace with life) in the older adult years.

Several life demands converge during adolescence. The adolescent must achieve a sense of healthy separation from his parents—inner and outer independence. This requires cutting inner dependency ties—a difficult, scary assignment, but absolutely essential if he is to emerge as a full person in his own right and sight. (Parents are often disturbed by the normal withdrawal of their teen-agers which is necessary for private growing.) The adolescent is also wrestling with powerful sexual feelings and fantasies, as a result of the physical maturity of the sex glands in puberty. Guilt feelings and excessive shyness often result from his inner struggles with blossoming sexuality. His sexual identity must be firmed up whether or not he is ready. Crucial and hard-to-reverse life decisions may be pushed on him by social expectations (communicated via parents, teachers

Understanding the Stages of Normal Development

and the draft). Choices of vocation, educational plans, life mate, and life philosophy—all of these decisions confront him while he is still struggling to discover who he really is. The way he decides in these choices will have a powerful impact on his eventual sense of self. Some youth "drop out," take a moratorium, to "find themselves" during middle or late adolescence. In the long run this may be better than making crucial decisions prematurely and unwisely. During early adolescence, the attraction to the opposite-sexed parent is revived. Parents and youth may defend themselves against awareness of their mutual attraction by conflict and rejection. In normal development, these reactivated feelings are transferred to peers of the opposite sex, and eventually to one in marriage.

The normal problems of adolescence are exaggerated and compounded in a period of lightning-fast social change such as ours. The chasm between the world in which the parents grew up and the world of the teen-ager is wide indeed. The models of maleness/femaleness and parenting absorbed by teens from their parents must be reshaped drastically to be useful in the new world of relationships that is emerging. Parents in their middle years also feel a wide gap between themselves and their senior citizen parents who often become emotionally dependent on their middle-aged "children." With gaps on both sides, parents are anxious and relationships difficult.

The adolescent who asks himself, "Do I really want to be like the square society of my parents?" is searching for an acceptable model of how to become a young adult. Models to which an adolescent can respond with enthusiasm are hard to come by in our present society with its wide generation chasms and its assassination of youth heroes. "Straight," boxed-in adults living driven, status-oriented existences can't expect to attract life-seeking adolescents to join them on their treadmill. Lacking attractive or relevant patterns of how others have handled the next stage in the journey of growth, one is forced to launch out on his own—without a map or a compass—and this is really scary business! Is it any wonder some young people prefer not to make the commitments (vocation, marriage, "settling down," economic self-sufficiency) which constitute the doorway to adulthood in our society?

Understanding the Stages of Normal Development

Many parents, teachers, and counselors are frustrated by their inability to connect with those young people who are disillusioned with the adult "establishment" values. The only hope of communication between these two groups is to start by recognizing the radical difference in the values affirmed by each.[4] Adults value production; these youth value pleasure as an end in itself. Vivid, here-and-now experience is valued by the youth who reject adult values such as success, achievement, disciplined development of skills. Peace and love are high values for the youth; aggressiveness and acquisitiveness are rejected as qualities leading to violence and exploitation. Instead of the adult valuing of safety, security and restraint, youth value risk, excitement and adventure. Mystical peak experiences are valued over the rationality and control by reason seen by adults as valuable. The authority-centered approaches to ethics are replaced by the youth's emphasis on love as the only necessary norm. The emphasis on the value of experiencing, pleasure, love, and peak experiences, makes for a whole new and freer approach to sex on the part of many young people, an area which is particularly distressing to parents who view the new morality of youth as immorality. It is worth noting that there is an intense ethical concern present in many youth in the "way out" group. They feel a deep revulsion at the world of adults which they see as a world of war, economic exploitation, depersonalization, racism, and sexual hypocrisy. Their urgent efforts to change these injustices are impressive. Their concerns face our society with the urgency of finding a new ethical sensitivity with respect to interpersonal values.

At each age and stage of their child's growth, parents experience themselves differently. They relive, often without realizing it, their own comparable growth stage. Old, unfinished inner conflicts from their adolescence, for example, may interfere with relating well with their teen-ager. They may unwittingly try to live out their unlived lives through their child. This reliving process can become a constructive thing, giving parents a second chance to do unfinished growth work with their "inner child of the past." This happens

---

4. We are indebted to Paul Pretzel's paper on "Whales and Polar Bears" for this conception of the radical value contrast between the two cultures.

only if they are aware of what is happening and make the necessary effort, perhaps with an assist from a professional counselor. Looking at why your child at a certain age makes you unreasonably out of sorts, anxious, or overprotective, can be productive. A child's growth phases and struggles are really an invitation to continuing growth on the part of his parents!

A skilled counselor can be a godsend when a child or youth is negotiating a difficult transition period, even if his services are not absolutely essential. The old idea that "only the sick need psychotherapeutic help" is out! Current thinking recognizes the fact that brief, well-timed professional help can speed up growth and help reduce the pain of a new, baffling life stage. A good counselor can help parents and their offspring use their own inner resources more fully, and thus cope constructively with a rough place on the developmental road. If a child or youth seems to be stuck at an earlier life task and stage, professional help is essential as a means of freeing him for continued growth.

Recommended Reading

Baruch, Dorothy W., *How to Live with Your Teen-Ager* (New York: McGraw-Hill Book Co., 1953) and *New Ways in Sex Education* (New York: McGraw-Hill Book Co., 1959). Practical guides.

Missildine, W. Hugh, *Your Inner Child of the Past* (New York: Simon & Schuster, 1963).

For helpful pamphlets on children and youth:

Public Affairs Pamphlets, 381 Park Avenue South, New York, New York 10016, and Child Study Association of America, 9 East 89th Street, New York, New York 10028.

4.

Finding Help

Suppose you have decided to find professional help, or at least some guidance in deciding whether it's needed. How do you go about finding such assistance? Where do you turn first? How do you know whether an individual or agency is professionally qualified and competent? How much will it cost? How long will it take?

Much depends on where you live. If you are in a city, there probably are many helping persons and agencies. But in a small town or rural area, your efforts to find help may be complicated by long distances to available resources.

Sources of Reliable Information

How do you discover what helping agencies and professionals are available in your community? Talk with someone you trust who knows the community well, or can find out what's available. A clergyman is often such a person. He probably has referred people to appropriate services frequently. If he's new in the area, he probably knows how to get reliable information from other professionals and social service directories. He can help you evaluate your need for help, and also suggest which services will meet your need. He'll probably know how to help you check on the training and credentials of private practitioners.

There are listings of helping agencies in many areas. Larger cities and counties often have directories of social service agencies, including

Finding Help

counseling facilities. Some have telephone information and referral services. Usually a call to the nearest office of the United Fund (or Community Chest), department of mental health, mental health association, or county welfare office, will either produce information about available agencies or tell you where to obtain it. Or, a letter to the national office of groups like The Family Service Association of America (44 East 23rd Street, New York, New York 10010), American Association of Marriage and Family Counselors (6211 West Northwest Highway, Dallas, Texas 75219), or The American Association of Pastoral Counselors (201 East 19th Street, New York, New York 10003), will get information regarding the nearest treatment agencies. Information about the training of professionals in private practice who treat children, youth, and families can usually be obtained by writing the national, state or local office of the appropriate professional association of the particular counseling discipline: pastoral counseling, social work, clinical psychology, psychiatry, marriage counseling.

How do you evaluate the professional competence of an agency or private practitioner? There are persons with inadequate training (including a few outright charlatans) in the field of counseling; care on this is important. Here are some of the questions to ask in evaluating a public or private nonprofit agency: Is its reputation good in the community? (No agency or individual enjoys everyone's approval, but community opinion should be generally positive if they're doing a competent job.) What do other professionals in the helping field think of it? (Check with your minister or doctor.) Is it funded by the United Fund or the Government or a body which holds member agencies accountable for accepted standards of practice? Is the agency administratively responsible to a board of citizens? Are you treated with respect by the agency personnel?

Evaluating those in private practice is difficult. Reputation is important, but it's no guarantee that the person is well trained. It is never out of place to ask either the person or the professional body which accredits him, what his training is for the job he's doing. If a professional person responds defensively, this in itself raises questions about the adequacy of his training. Be especially careful when

Finding Help

considering help from a "marriage counselor"; check to make sure he is well trained.

Not all psychologists, social workers, psychiatrists, and clergymen are trained as counselors. Clinical and counseling psychologists are so trained, as are counseling social workers. Psychiatrists who specialize in neurology may not be competent psychotherapists. Most nonpsychiatric physicians and lawyers have had little or no training in counseling on emotional problems, although they may know about reliable referral resources. Clergymen not specializing in counseling often have had sufficient training in counseling to equip them to recognize severe problems, make appropriate referrals, and engage in brief crisis counseling and marriage counseling in less severe problems. Some doctors are aware enough of psychological factors to help parents decide whether counseling is needed. Much depends on the clergyman's or doctor's sensitivity and openness to the complex realm of relationships.

It is sometimes helpful to talk with more than one agency or counselor before deciding on which to try. Find a counselor in whom you can develop confidence. If this confidence is not established within a reasonable period of time it is important to discuss your feelings with the counselor; if the block continues it is quite legitimate to end the relationship and try another counselor or agency. However, if you find yourself "shopping around" regularly or often, then you should begin to wonder whether your resistance to change is interfering.

How much will counseling cost? This varies according to the helping person or agency. Private practitioners usually charge considerably more than agencies. Agencies supported by taxes or community funds use sliding fee scales based on the family's amount of income in relation to the number of people dependent on it. If you're considering help from a private practitioner, check on going rates in your community for persons of that particular training and experience. Whenever you get help, be sure to have a clear, mutually acceptable understanding of precisely what the fee will be. (As a person who cares about people and your community, you may well decide to join forces with those groups who are attempting to

Finding Help

provide more services, especially for troubled children, on an ability-to-pay basis. This is an area in which churches should be involved through their social action committees.)

How long will the counseling be needed? The answer varies with the nature and severity of the problem. Occasionally, one or two sessions can clarify things enough that the family or couple can take it from there. It is wise to commit yourself to at least a half dozen sessions before you decide whether to continue. Many people become discouraged around the third or fourth sessions and drop out before they've really discovered if it could help them. Often at least two or three months are required. Some change should be noted by this time if the counseling is effective. Some people continue in therapy for many months. This is sometimes necessary if the problems are severe or if a person or family is living under continual stress. Some of the newer crisis counseling approaches, however, can often shorten the time needed for relatively healthy families to make real progress in mobilizing their latent strengths, improving their communication, and pulling out of the tailspin of their crisis.

After regular sessions are over, many counselors encourage people to check back occasionally or to get in touch whenever they feel the need to talk things over. You should feel free to use this kind of professional help in much the same way that you use dental or medical checkups—to get help with minor problems and to prevent future trouble.

What to Tell Your Child

How should you explain the need for help to your child once you have decided to seek it? It is always best to tell the truth: "This family has some problems and we are all going to get some help in figuring them out," or "We have all been unhappy lately and we are going to see whether we can get some help to make things better."

"We are worried about the fact that you are having trouble at school (unhappy, having bad dreams, setting fires, using drugs, running away), and we are going to see whether we can get some help with the problem."

Finding Help

It's well to avoid making the child feel that he is the only problem, even if he is the one with obvious symptoms. He will be more responsive to therapy if he feels his parents or family recognize their own problems and involvement. Thus it would not be wise to say: "You have been misbehaving lately and we are going to take you to a counselor," or "Your teacher says you are not getting along in school and you need some help."

Emphasis on the "we" aspect of the situation takes some of the burden of responsibility for change off the child and spreads it around in the family where it actually belongs.

Don't offer the child a choice about going to the counselor unless you really mean for it to be his choice. "Would you like for us to go and get some help with this problem?" often brings a "No!" Then you are faced with talking him into it, or forcing him, if that doesn't work. It is usually better to make a positive statement that "we are going" with the assumption that he will accept your judgment as he does in most other things.

Of course, the age of the child influences how you present the idea. A small child need only be informed of the plans and helped to deal with his feelings about it. An older child may take some part in the discussion providing the parents retain the final decision. With adolescents, it's a different story. It's rarely productive to insist that a young person get help if he resists strongly. The parents can present the problem as a family one; often the adolescent will respond positively enough to give it a try at least.

What if a child or adolescent objects or refuses to come? If it's a younger child it would be handled in the same way you handle other things he has to do but doesn't want to: "I know you don't like the idea but we are going to give it a try and see if it helps us all feel better." Accepting and understanding his fears, while at the same time assuming that it must be done, is usually best. Getting into verbal battles sabotages the experience in advance. The child feels forced to get nothing from counseling, in order to win the battle against his parents. If the child continues resisting once he has begun coming, it is the counselor's job to help with the feelings

Finding Help

and to decide along with the parents whether to continue or to try some other course.

With an adolescent who isn't interested or strongly resists, it is usually best for the parents to get help themselves in the hope that changing their approach to him will alleviate the problem or that he will decide on his own to get help. Sometimes it is possible to insist on "giving it a try" for one or more sessions with the understanding that he may terminate if he doesn't like it. A counselor who relates well to adolescents can often "get through to them" when parents can't, simply because adolescents need to fight their parents as part of the process of becoming free to grow up. Sometimes an adult outside the family—a teacher, pastor or school counselor—can motivate a youth to get counseling help when the parents can't.

It is never a good idea to try to fool children about the reason for getting help. They always know it isn't just for fun. They are entitled to an explanation appropriate to their age. They may not be ready to accept the explanation, or able to understand it fully, but they need to know what the adults involved have in mind.

What Will It Be Like?

Even when you decide that it's necessary, it is hard to ask for help. As parents, we feel we should know how to raise our children, make them happy, and avoid problems. When anything goes wrong, we feel we have somehow failed. This book has been emphasizing the importance of remembering that we're human and therefore we often make mistakes and fail to measure up to our own goals as parents. This does not mean we have failed as persons. As Alfred Adler once said, we need "the courage of our imperfections." Everyone needs help at times; many of us muddle through without it but we'd do a lot better if we had it. Actually it's a sign of strength to be able to say "Yes, something has gone wrong. We need help." (If you and your spouse can't agree on the need for help, the one who feels assistance is needed should have a few ses-

Finding Help

sions with a counselor to evaluate the need and decide if he wishes to get help with his side of the relationship.)

A counselor often enlists the parents' help even before he sees the child. He usually wants to know two kinds of things: factual information about the child, and what the emotional climate of the home is like—its positive resources and its problems. The first interview with the parents is their opportunity to assess the counselor as well, to talk over their fears and feelings with him and to sense his potential helpfulness. Parents should discuss openly with the counselor any negative feelings they may have in this initial contact. (Some counselors want to see the whole family the first time. They feel that they can assess the situation more fully and be more helpful in their recommendations if they begin this way. Either method can be effective. Which one is used usually depends on the individual counselor's particular preferences and the nature of the problem.)

Feelings of uneasiness and guilt which often remain after one begins counseling may interfere with the helping relationship. As parents we don't like the feeling that someone else can succeed where we believe we have failed. When your child begins to change in counseling you may feel it is further evidence that it is "all our fault." Many parents withdraw their children and themselves when the child begins to change.

Actually, when a child improves, it's usually because the whole family has changed, not because of some magic the counselor has worked. If your child stays improved, it has to be to your credit as well as the therapist's skill.

Watch for unconscious resistance to change. Whatever took you to counseling was painful enough for you to want help; but you may feel uneasy when things start to become really different. The way things were was at least familiar. Who knows what a different way may be like? Will it be better? Or worse? Will future satisfactions make the present struggles to change family relationships worthwhile? Let's face it, change is hard work.

In counseling, things often get worse before they get better. Since things were already bad, you probably feel you really can't stand it if they get worse. It helps to know that this is an expected phase and is temporary. A seriously misbehaving child may become more difficult after several sessions of play therapy. Sometimes it's because he's learning new ways to deal with feelings and isn't very good at it yet. Sometimes it's his own resistance to change; sometimes he's testing out his parents to see whether they really mean their new approach. Usually such a regression passes if parents can be patient enough, long enough.

It is easy for parents to feel left out, or angry, or doubtful about the value of it when their child is involved in counseling. This is particularly true if the parents are not themselves involved in counseling or if they are seeing a different counselor. They may have little contact with the child's counselor. But it also happens when the same person is working with both parents and child. Parents have a right and responsibility to make as sure as they can of the counselor's competence and the effectiveness of his therapy. If they have reservations they should be certain to bring them into the open where they can be discussed and resolved if possible, before they decide to give up the process. Sometimes such a discussion actually helps the therapy to progress more rapidly.

Parents are often bothered by the confidential nature of what goes on between child and counselor. They feel they have a right to know what happens. Child counselors, however, insist on confidentiality for many reasons. They feel it shows respect for the child and encourages him to trust the therapist with his inmost fears and feelings. This trust cannot develop if the child suspects that his words or actions may be reported to his parents.

It is almost inevitable, and is certainly very human, that parents will be angry at their child's counselor at times. They have a right to be. But for this reason, it is all the more vital that they be able to trust the counselor both with their child, and with their angry and mixed up feelings about the counseling. The anger will cause trouble only if they are not aware of it or if they do not deal with it directly in conversation with their own or the child's counselor.

Parents sometimes sabotage the child's therapy without realizing it if they are unaware of their negative feelings. Bringing a child

Finding Help

late to his sessions, cancelling them at the drop of a hat, making the child feel guilty about the money being spent, undermining the child's confidence in the counselor, are all subtle ways of sabotage. When parents are also seeing a counselor regularly they can deal with their feelings openly so that the sabotage is less likely to occur. A good counselor will encourage them to do this.

Usually change does not happen fast enough to suit us when we're hurting. You may feel that you have improved as parents, but your child is going right on with his perverse ways. Try to bear with it. Patience is a major ingredient of successful therapy. You can't expect to undo in a few weeks what has been developing over many years. Also, children often wait until they are sure the family situation is different before they show changes that are taking place in themselves.

Between counseling sessions, families should try out their new ways of communication. Often, in the beginning, they don't work. Or newly discovered feelings stirred up in counseling come popping out at home in hurting ways. These things are discouraging.

It helps for parents to work on increasing the satisfactions in their marriage. This relieves the pressure of impatience for the child to change, and increases the security of the family so that it is safer for everyone to change. Dealing with our own stress, independent of our children, relieves the burden for everyone. Plan and do some things as a couple. Don't wait till the child improves to have some fun yourselves. He or she will improve faster if you let yourselves enjoy being a man and a woman sharing each other and life.

Sometimes parents feel that they should be able to solve their own and their child's problems by the use of religious practices such as individual and family prayer, Bible reading, and devotions. They believe that having to ask for the help of a counselor is somehow an admission of failure in their religion. But God is the spirit of life and growth and can work through a skilled counselor (whether or not that person uses "religious" language). He may help free the family to "live its religion" more fully in their relationships. As communication and relationships improve within the family, religious practices may, for some, be meaningful ways of

Finding Help

expressing and celebrating new joy, honesty, vitality, and unity within the family.

To continue the growth impetus of counseling, join a growth group for parents. This is a small (twelve or less) group designed to stimulate the rate of normal growth in reasonably healthy people. The gains you've made in counseling will be more likely to continue and expand as you want them to, if you don't try to "go it alone." By meeting regularly with other parents who also want to improve their marriages and families, you can be helpful to each other.

If no group exists, start one! The leader should be trained in facilitating communication in small groups. Your clergyman may have this training or know someone who does. Growth groups (in contrast to most other groups) encourage honest sharing and mutual caring. (You can encourage your church to become a more exciting place by helping to develop a network of growth groups, for persons at all the life stages. Such groups are the ideal method for a church that wants to be true to its mission—that of becoming a center of healing, and growth and training for helping others.)

The continuing growth of your family can be nourished by participating in the church and community organizations (YMCA, adult education, scouts, service groups which you find meaningful. Avoid the danger of overinvolvement (which can hurt families) but keep connected with those groups which provide enjoyable relationships, broadening of your horizons, and opportunity to make your community a better place for people! Particularly important is the cultivation of a supportive circle of friends and/or relatives, to be your "extended family"—your support group or spiritual clan. Such a circle is vital to family emotional health, especially during periods of crisis.

After Help

If you find a competent counselor and work hard at changing, you'll learn new skills in relating and communicating. You will need the counselor less and less as you employ these skills in im-

Finding Help

proving your family relationships. ("Improving" means making them more mutually satisfying.) An unhappy relationship isn't like a broken leg that can be taken for granted once it's healed. It's more like a muscle weakened through long disuse; continuing exercise is essential to keeping it healthy. The value of counseling isn't that of getting a disturbed child or relationship "fixed"; the real value is in the new skills your family acquires to keep everyone in the family "going and growing." It takes continuing effort, but counseling lets you discover both that you can do it and how.

The grooves of old relationship patterns are deep; it's easy to slip back into them. There is a strange attraction in old, familiar ruts; only the new satisfactions of better, closer relating can keep you from backsliding. When you feel your relationships slipping, use what you have learned in counseling—talk about it in the family and decide what needs to be done to get off the skids. If this doesn't help, arrange quickly for a few "retread" counseling sessions to help you get back on the growth track.

Recommended Reading

Clinebell, H. J., Jr., and Charlotte H., *The Intimate Marriage* (New York: Harper & Row, 1970).

Halpern, H. M., *A Parent's Guide to Child Psychotherapy* (New York: A. S. Barnes and Co., 1963). Discusses the role of parents.

Moustakas, Clark E., *Psychotherapy with Children* (New York: Harper & Row, 1959). Includes a chapter on parents' use of play therapy to help children deal with crises.

5.

Coping with Family Crises

A crisis happens within a person (or family) rather than simply to him. Difficult circumstances such as prolonged illness, the birth of a handicapped child, a divorce, an accident, or a death are a part of nearly everyone's experience. Our response to the emergency or the difficulty determines whether or not the crisis will be a growth experience. There are several principles which we have found can be helpful in handling crises constructively:

1) Your response to a crisis-inducing situation is within your control. How an individual responds to difficult circumstances depends on many things within him—his philosophy of life; his relationships; coping abilities he has developed previously; other stresses and satisfactions; religious and emotional resources. A young mother commented, "Realizing that we could choose how we reacted to the blow of having to pull up our roots and move gave us a feeling of strength along with our pain."

2) Face and express the big feelings that accompany every crisis. Feelings of loss, anger, guilt, resentment, confusion, helplessness, despair and even temporary disorientation, panic, and paralysis are often a part of the first response to a crisis-inducing situation. These feelings must be dealt with so that your coping abilities can be used creatively. Weeping, talking out painful feelings with an empathetic person—spouse, friend, clergyman, counselor—are ways

Coping with Family Crises

of working through the painful feelings. Children should be encouraged to talk out and play out their fear and hurt. Four-year-old Joel played "wreck" for several months after a family automobile accident, crashing his toy cars into each other violently as he relived and resolved painful memories. Burdensome feelings openly dealt with gradually diminish, freeing you to use your mind more efficiently in handling the external difficulties. Stored up, they only cripple your ability to act constructively.

3) Accept the fact that crises and living go together. Of course there are bound to be feelings of hurt and anger when life treats you harshly. But if you can avoid getting stuck in resentment and guilt (Why did this happen to me? or, I must have done something bad to deserve this), you will be able to take appropriate action sooner. Self-pity is an expensive luxury. The person (or family) who gets mired down in it doesn't have incentive or energy left for dealing with the crisis.

4) Decide on some positive action, however small. The personality is like a muscle—using it to improve your situation makes it stronger and healthier. Exercising your coping abilities by standing off (perhaps with a counselor's help) and getting an overview of the situation, then deciding on one option, and moving into action, usually makes you feel less helpless. Taking action does not necessarily mean you can change the external situation. Losing a loved one through death is something that cannot be changed. But you can do something that will strengthen you to cope with the tremendous loss.

5) Turn toward people. Don't be afraid to lean on them. Many people experiencing a crisis are tempted to isolate themselves from others, because of loneliness, or the mistaken notion that stoic self-sufficiency is a virtue, or because they fear they will be a burden to others. But people need people and people need to be needed. A crisis occurs within us when important foods of the spirit, such as acceptance, belonging, caring, devotion, esteem, faith, are threatened or cut off. The loss of a loving relationship, an esteem-feeding job, financial security, dreams for one's children, a house that feels like home, a healthy body, the life stage one has gotten used to,

Coping with Family Crises

means there probably will be a crisis within. Withdrawing from people only intensifies the loss. (It also deprives others of the chance to be needed.) Temporary sources of nourishment in helpful relationships give one strength to handle losses. Replacing lost emotional nurturance by developing new relationships is essential for long-range recovery. In the acute stages of crisis, a few sessions with a skilled counselor can be extremely helpful in recovering from the staggering blow and mobilizing your own resources.

6) Remember that coping successfully with a crisis actually makes you stronger. A crisis is like a fork in the road, one moves in the right direction or the wrong—toward either weakening or strengthening his coping abilities. Each crisis, if it is handled constructively, leaves you better equipped for the next one. A family which lives through and handles painful problems together without collapsing is bound together in new strength and closeness. After his nine-year-old son's serious accident, one father said, "Terry's hospitalization forced us to pull together as a family. We found out we have guts when it counts." An unexpected fringe benefit of crisis is that a person or family discovers unused inner resources.

7) Let yourself lean on the Eternal—on God. Don't be afraid to ask the big questions which the crisis within you stirs. A crisis forces us to draw on all our spiritual resources. What does it all mean? How does it fit into our family's philosophy of living? Are our values workable when the going gets tough? What value changes do we need to make in response to the new awareness of how brief, fragile and precious our life together is?

A doctor in California asks his nearly recovered heart patients, "What have you learned from this experience?" This is an appropriate question once one is beginning to get on top of things again. Not to ask it is to waste the opportunity for spiritual growth. The wife of a recovering alcoholic said, "We didn't expect to get reconnected with a higher Power and to rejoin the human race as a result of Ben's alcoholism, but that's just what happened to us in AA and Al-Anon." If your religious beliefs and experiences let you know the reality of "leaning on the everlasting arms," you have an invaluable strength for crisis. This spiritual strength can be in-

Coping with Family Crises

creased through the soul-searching opportunities of a crisis. Talking over the deep questions of faith and values with a theologically trained counselor (your minister, priest, or rabbi) can help to stimulate this growth in the vertical dimension of your family and personal life.

Holding these principles of constructive coping in mind, let's look at several specific problems faced by tens of thousands of parents.

The Handicapped Child

If your child is physically handicapped or mentally retarded your situation is continually demanding, discouraging, and frustrating. Someone has described parents of a permanently handicapped child as living with chronic grief, a dark cloud always hanging somewhere in their consciousness. Here are some guidelines which may be helpful:

First, it is crucial to deal candidly with your feelings; discuss them often with your spouse. If yours is a one-parent family, find a caring adult with whom to talk through your pain. Parents of handicapped children experience a whirl of feelings—resentment, confusion, disappointment, shame, grief, and guilt, combined with tenderness, protectiveness, and intense caring. Feelings that aren't "owned" or recognized interfere with a parent's relationship with his handicapped child. Hidden resentment toward one's spouse, in handicaps which may have some basis in heredity, inhibits marital intimacy. If you can't talk out your painful feelings thoroughly with each other, get professional assistance.

Second, find the best diagnostic treatment and rehabilitation services available to you. The vast majority of handicapped persons can achieve a satisfying and relatively self-sufficient life. The therapy may be long, but the alternative is a life of dependent futility. Get your doctor's and clergyman's advice about local helping agencies and financial assistance. With this information in hand, take action! Long delays may make rehabilitation more difficult.

Third, do everything you can to avoid treating your child as special. Overprotecting and pampering him seem kind now, but they will prove to be "cruel kindness," denying him the learning-through-

Coping with Family Crises

struggle that produces that degree of mastery of which he is capable. Of course it is important to recognize his actual limitations and avoid unrealistic expectations which only frustrate him and you. But normal parental reflexes make you want to "help" your handicapped child more than is really helpful. The guideline is: don't do anything for him that he may be able to learn to do for himself if he has to.

Fourth, learn to accept your child the way he is. This is hard advice, for it is difficult to distinguish realistic from unrealistic expectations. All parents have dreams and aspirations for their children. Parents of a handicapped child are forced to revise or relinquish these. It is harder for everyone if the parents continue to hope for the miracle rather than accepting the child's worth as he is.

Fifth, encourage your child to talk out and play out his own feelings. His self-image will be colored by his unresolved conflicts and fantasies about his body, as well as his perception of how you really feel about him. If you have other children, they should also have opportunities to talk or play through their feelings—jealousy about special treatment of him, nonrational guilt about being unhandicapped, a sense of family stigma. A child or family therapist may be necessary to help you all get at half-buried feelings.

Finally, relinquish inappropriate self-blame and the theological distortions which cause some parents to feel (even though they don't really believe it) that God or life is punishing them for some known or unknown sin. Such punitive, unflattering pictures of God certainly don't fit the best understandings of him in our religious heritage. A clinically trained clergyman is often the best-equipped person to help you deal with such theological distortions, and achieve the positive spiritual perspective needed to carry a heavy load.

Prolonged Illnesses

Long illness, particularly if it involves hospitalization, can leave unhealed emotional wounds. Separation from security-giving relationships, strange, threatening surroundings, and the anxiety, boredom and pain, often make hospitalizations traumatic to children.

Coping with Family Crises

Parents of young children should insist on being with them. After an upsetting experience at a hospital or doctor's office, create an opportunity for your child or youth to talk about his feelings and fantasies (often of death or the loss of a part of his body). Homegrown or professional play therapy can be invaluable; let young children play out their anger and fear, for example by sticking a needle in a doll representing the doctor or the nurse. As in other problems, the rule is the same—don't let the painful feelings lie buried and festering.

The other troublesome result of prolonged illness is missing important learning experiences. Jill was hospitalized with rheumatic fever during what should have been her freshman year in high school. A home teacher supplied by the school helped her keep up academically. What she missed was a year of learning new social skills—things like how to talk with boys—which her peers were busily practicing. Having fallen behind, it was difficult to catch up; since she was both shy and socially inept, she continued to fail in social situations. Some coaching and encouragement in a small support group (a teen self-discovery group with a trained adult leader in her church) were necessary to help Jill get back in stride with her age group.

Drug Problems

Many teen-agers and pre-teens are involved in the "drug scene." This is particularly frightening to parents for whom it conjures up visions of drug addiction, delinquency, and sexual problems. Like all human problems, this one is complex. Youth use drugs for many different reasons and in ways that involve danger from little to very great. Unfortunately, parental panic reactions tend to lump all drug use together. Some youth (and adults) use drugs to deaden terrible psychological pain or to opt out of grim external reality—ghettoes, war, pollution, overpopulation. For these, drug use is more a case of turning off than turning on. But thousands of youth dabble in drug use, particularly "pot," to share in a peer-group ritual, for a "peak experience," or simply to try something exciting of which the square adult world vigorously disapproves. The vast majority of this group will probably experience no lasting harmful effects, although there's always risk—a fact which makes drug use more rather than less attractive to most youth. Only a small percentage of marijuana users, according to recent research, move on to heroin addiction.

Here are some suggestions which may help if you know or suspect that your teen-ager is using drugs. (The same approach applies if he is involved in sexual activities of which you disapprove.)

First, don't panic! If you're "up tight" about drugs, talk to a counselor who can help you get the problem in perspective before you try to discuss it with your son or daughter. Otherwise, you may wreck communication between you just when it is most needed. A counselor who understands the youth counterculture can help you decide what course of action or inaction will probably contribute to your teen-ager's real safety and growth toward adulthood, and not simply shatter what may already be a shaky relationship between you.

Second, don't exaggerate or use heavy-handed methods. If your parents used such methods with you as an adolescent, you can probably still remember your fury, hurt and resentment. Heavy-handed methods of discipline simply don't work, and they usually backfire, especially with teen-agers. Teens are expert at making tyrants feel guilty. Harsh external discipline delays rather than fosters the emergence of what the adolescent must develop to be a responsible adult—*self*-discipline. Most important, heavy-handedness tends to weaken or destroy the most precious thing of all—your relationship. Your son or daughter needs that, even if he doesn't show it; so do you! Parental overreacting to superficial experimentation with drugs may make it continue as a way of rebelliously establishing one's separate identity.

Third, continue to set limits but only on things that are really important and are enforceable. Don't waste your parental influence on things like length of hair, which is a powerful symbol of peer-group identity and the strength of youth to defy the establishment. If you spend your influence trying to get your youth to conform to adult standards for hair and clothes, you probably won't have any left for things like respect, integrity and love.

Fourth, keep working at strengthening the lines of communication. If they're broken and you can't repair them, get the help of a

Coping with Family Crises

family counselor, who is trained as a communications facilitator. There are periods during the teens when a youth cuts communication from his end, much of the time. He needs to live in his world to do his own private growing and discovering of himself. When this happens, stay available but don't try to force your way into his world. Incidentally, the ability of your child or youth to communicate negative feelings toward you and articulate vigorous disagreements, probably is a sign that you have succeeded in giving him enough room to become himself.

Fifth, set a positive example of the *responsible* use or non-use of drugs (alcohol, nicotine, sleeping pills). Example is still the most powerful teacher. "Thou shalt nots" are singularly unconvincing to youth, particularly if parents are also misusing their own favorite consciousness-altering drugs. The real issue in the use/misuse of a given drug is, "How much and under what circumstances does its use enhance or diminish the life of the user and his relationships?" Responsible use means using any drug only in those situations and amounts which keep the danger of hurting persons at an absolute minimum. Responsible non-use of any drug means abstaining in ways that neither "drives others to drink," nor rejects judgmentally the possible benefits of their use by others. In our drug-saturated culture, learning what responsible behavior and attitudes are, relative to drugs, is a vital part of the preparation of children and youth for constructive adulthood.

Sixth, make therapy available for your teen-ager, if you know that he is in real trouble with drugs or that his use of them is symptomatic of deep unhappiness. Many cities now have free clinics where youth can get medical and counseling help, on a walk-in basis, without parental consent and even without giving their names. Your city should have such an easily available service tailored especially to rebelling, alienated youth. Telephone crisis clinics (sometimes called "hot line" services) with a special emphasis on helping drug users, are also valuable community resources. Some churches are taking the initiative and cooperating in such projects.

Above all, develop a life style that includes genuine excitement about living, the only long-range, positive alternative to drug use.

Coping with Family Crises

As one high school girl put it, after she had found this life style in a growth group led by her minister, "I'm really turned on to nature, books, music, and most all, people! It's beautiful!" In a word, if the job of the family and of the church is to help persons of all ages find "life in all its fullness," these institutions are key instruments for preventing drug abuse.

One-Parent Families

The millions of parents who must be both mother and father have a demanding, but not impossible, assignment. Here are some ways of handling the pressures constructively.

First, build a support group—a set of relationships with other adults and families to meet your needs for adult companionship and your child's need for relationships with adults of both sexes. Two likely places to meet compatible friends are in neighborhood churches and groups like Parents Without Partners. There's a lot of giving involved in being a parent, and even more in being a double-parent. A child gives much in return, but it's not the same as what one gets and needs from nurturing adults. If we try to get adult-type satisfactions from our children, they may feel resentful or deprived of their childhood. A close relationship with at least one caring adult is essential to your own emotional vitality and parental adequacy.

A child needs closeness to adults of both sexes as he forms his own sense of identity. If you're a single parent because of divorce, give your children ample opportunity to continue or increase their relationship with your ex-spouse. However you feel about him he is still immensely important psychologically to the child you co-created. It is important that children feel they can love both parents, without losing the love of either one. Children should never be pawns which each divorced parent uses against the other. If death caused your singleness, it may be more difficult to provide ample relationships for your child with one or more caring people of the opposite sex. Arranging for such relating is one of the important things you can do to help your child cope with the loss of a parent.

It is most important what you do with your feelings about your

Coping with Family Crises

singleness—resentment, regret, wounded self-esteem, grief, loneliness, sexual frustration or guilt, and rejection. In a society that makes two-parent families the norm, one-parent families often feel inferior or even abnormal, which only compounds the reality problems of maintaining a growth-fostering family climate. If you find yourself stewing regularly in your feelings, obtain counseling to help you resolve the inner conflicts that are reducing your enjoyment of life and your children. Remember the crucial thing for children in one *or* two-parent families is the quality of the parent-child relationship. That's what will make the difference in their lives; the quality of your relations with them is something you can improve.

Life is a series of crises, large and small, expected and unexpected. If we can help our children to "see that this thing which has happened to us, even though it may be a life-shaking experience, does not of necessity have to be a life-breaking one,"[1] they will be better able to handle crisis constructively.

Transmitting a Religious Orientation to Children

Many parents ask themselves, "How can we help our children to develop a religious orientation?" Often such parents are aware of the fact that external and conventional ways of doing this—attending church school and saying grace at meals, for example—are not in themselves adequate, unless something else is also present. This essential "something else" is a *certain quality of relationships in the family, within which the heart of constructive religion actually can be experienced.* If this quality of relationships is experienced, to some degree, part of the time, then a deep-level religious attitude toward persons and life will be caught by the children and reaffirmed in the adults. Having caught something of this heart-level experience and made it their own, children can then find meaning in the religious ideas and beliefs which they are taught on a head level. The possession of heart-level religious attitudes is a precious resource for meeting the misery and grandeur of life and for continuing to grow

1. The words of the parents of a mentally retarded child. Mrs. Max A. Murray, "Needs of Parents of Mentally Retarded Children," *American Journal of Mental Deficiency* (May 1959), p. 1084.

Coping with Family Crises

as a person, at each age and stage. A person who has reconciled and integrated his heart-level and head-level religion is best prepared to cope creatively with his painful and joyous experiences.

The quality of relationships in which religion becomes an experienced reality—allowing the family to "live its religion"—is the kind of accepting, nonjudgmental, caring, responsive and responsible relationships which are the theme of this volume. Let's look at the basic ingredients of a "religious orientation." These include: the feeling of deep trust and at-homeness inside oneself, with others, and in the universe; a fundamental respect for self, others, and nature; the ability and the inclination to give and receive love; a lively awareness of the wonder of the commonplace—awe in the presence of a new baby, a sunset, a friendship; a philosophy of life that makes sense and guides decisions toward responsible behavior; a dedication with enthusiasm to the larger good of persons and society.

What helps a child to incorporate these ingredients as a part of himself? The ability to trust (which is the heart of faith) grows in the warm, dependable, nurturing relationship of the infant with the mothering and fathering persons. The ability to accept, respect, and love others is a learned ability; it develops *only* in a relationship in which the child *receives* acceptance, respect, and love for what he is— a person of worth. This is the experience of grace—receiving the love one doesn't have to earn. This experience and the sure knowledge that one is loved and cared for, whatever happens, is the foundation for personal growth. It is the context which makes discipline— learning to know and cooperate with the rules of good relationships—effective in producing a responsible person. A maturing philosophy of life and workable values to guide one's decisions are the result of internalizing the values of one's family and then changing and refining them to make them genuinely one's own. A commitment to the larger good, a sense of wonder, and the ability to say "yes" to life and all it brings are caught by children who experience them in the need-satisfying adults in their early life. As is often painfully obvious to parents, children have an amazing awareness of our real life style, our real values, our real commitments—in short, our real religion. Frequently they take within themselves and mirror back to us in their behavior, not our head-level, Saturday or Sunday morning religion, but our deeper orientations of which *we* may not be fully aware until we see it in them. When this happens, it's a challenge to do some more work on the lifelong task of keeping our basic religious life growing.

Every crisis is a spiritual crisis and an opportunity for spiritual growth; it is a chance to reexamine our answers to the big questions of life—the questions with which our religious heritage has struggled through the centuries. Why do we suffer? What is life all about? What is worth living for? Sometimes we have trouble admitting to our children that we haven't got all the answers, although such an admission may be the stimulus that encourages them to search for their own meanings and values.

In the final analysis, the resources for using painful experiences creatively come from relationships—with oneself, with one's family and friends, and with God. In a world of uncertainty and insecurity, "things outside ourselves change—and many times we have little control over those elements—but if we learn to utilize our inner resources, we carry our security around with us."[2] The only certainty is that the future will be a surprise. We cannot avoid crisis, but learning to handle each one as it comes, and using it as a growth experience, makes us better prepared for the surprises of the future, and assures our children a chance of growing up as the independent and creative persons we dream for them to be.

2. Virginia M. Axline, *Dibs: In Search of Self* (Boston: Houghton Mifflin Co., 1965), p. 51.

Recommended Reading

Ayrault, Evelyn W., *You Can Raise Your Handicapped Child* (New York: G. P. Putnam's Sons, 1964). A guide for parents.

Melton, David, *Todd, A Father's Story* (New York: Dell Books, 1968). How a brain-injured boy was helped.